Delicious Air Fryer Poultry Dishes and Desserts

A Cooking Guide to Super Tasty, Easy and Affordable Air Fryer Poultry Meals and Desserts

By Donna Thomson

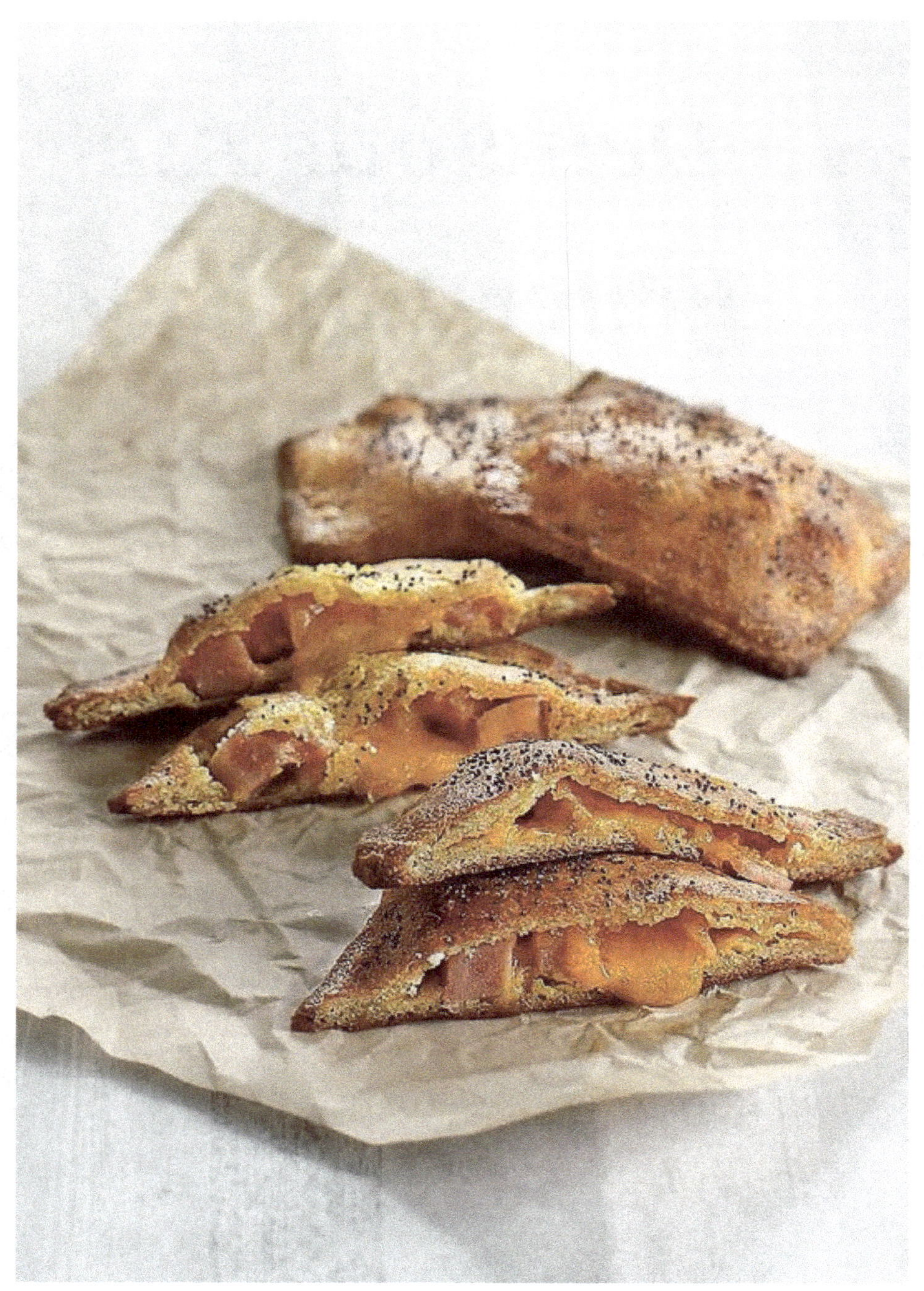

The content within this book has been derived from various sources. Please consult a licensed professional before attempting any techniques outlined in this book.

By reading this document, the reader agrees that under no circumstances is the author responsible for any losses, direct or indirect, which are incurred as a result of the use of information contained within this document, including, but not limited to, — errors, omissions, or inaccuracies.

Table of Contents

POULTRY 10

Spinach-Egg with Coconut Milk Casserole.......................... 11

Sriracha-Ginger Chicken...14

Sriracha-vinegar Marinated Chicken...............................16

Sticky-Sweet Chicken BBQ 19

Sweet Lime 'n Chili Chicken Barbecue 21

Teriyaki Glazed Chicken Bake 24

Tomato, Cheese 'n Broccoli Quiche 26

Tomato, Eggplant 'n Chicken Skewers 28

Turmeric and Lemongrass Chicken Roast.........................31

Apple Pie in Air Fryer..35

Apple-Toffee Upside-Down Cake 38

Banana-Choco Brownies.. 40

Blueberry & Lemon Cake 42

Bread Pudding with Cranberry...................................45

Cherries 'n Almond Flour Bars 46

Cherry-Choco Bars 48

Chocolate Chip inside a Mug 50

Choco-Peanut Mug Cake...52

Coco-Lime Bars 54

Coconut 'n Almond Fat Bombs 56

Coconutty Lemon Bars 57

Coffee 'n Blueberry Cake.. 60

Coffee Flavored Cookie Dough 62

Coffee Flavored Doughnuts 64

Crisped 'n Chewy Chonut Holes 66

Crispy Good Peaches... 69

Easy Baked Chocolate Mug Cake...................................... 71

Hot Coconut 'n Cocoa Buns 73

Keto-Friendly Doughnut Recipe 75

Lava Cake in A Mug..77

Leche Flan Filipino Style..79

Lusciously Easy Brownies 81

Maple Cinnamon Buns... 83

Melts in Your Mouth Caramel Cheesecake........................ 86

Mouth-Watering Strawberry Cobbler................................ 88

Oriental Coconut Cake 90

Pecan-Cranberry Cake 91

Poppy Seed Pound Cake... 93

Pound Cake with Fresh Apples 95

Quick 'n Easy Pumpkin Pie 97

Raspberry-Coco Desert 99

Raspberry-Coconut Cupcake 100

Strawberry Pop-Tarts...102

Strawberry Shortcake Quickie 105

Vanilla Pound Cake 107

Yummy Banana Cookies 108

Zucchini-Choco Bread.. 110

POULTRY

Spinach-Egg with Coconut Milk Casserole

Serves: 6

Cooking Time: 20 minutes

Ingredients:

- ¼ cup coconut milk /62.5ML
- 1 onion, chopped
- 1 teaspoon garlic powder /5G
- 12 large eggs, beaten
- 2 tablespoons coconut oil /30ML
- 3 cups spinach, chopped /390G
- Salt and pepper to taste

Instructions:

1) Preheat the air fryer for 5 minutes.
2) Combine all ingredients except the spinach in a mixing bowl. Whisk until well combined.
3) Place the spinach in a baking dish and pour the egg mixture
4) Place in mid-air fryer chamber and cook for 20 minutes at 310° F or 155°C .

Nutrition information:

- Calories per serving:185

- Carbohydrates: 3.2g
- Protein: 6.9g
- Fat: 16.1g

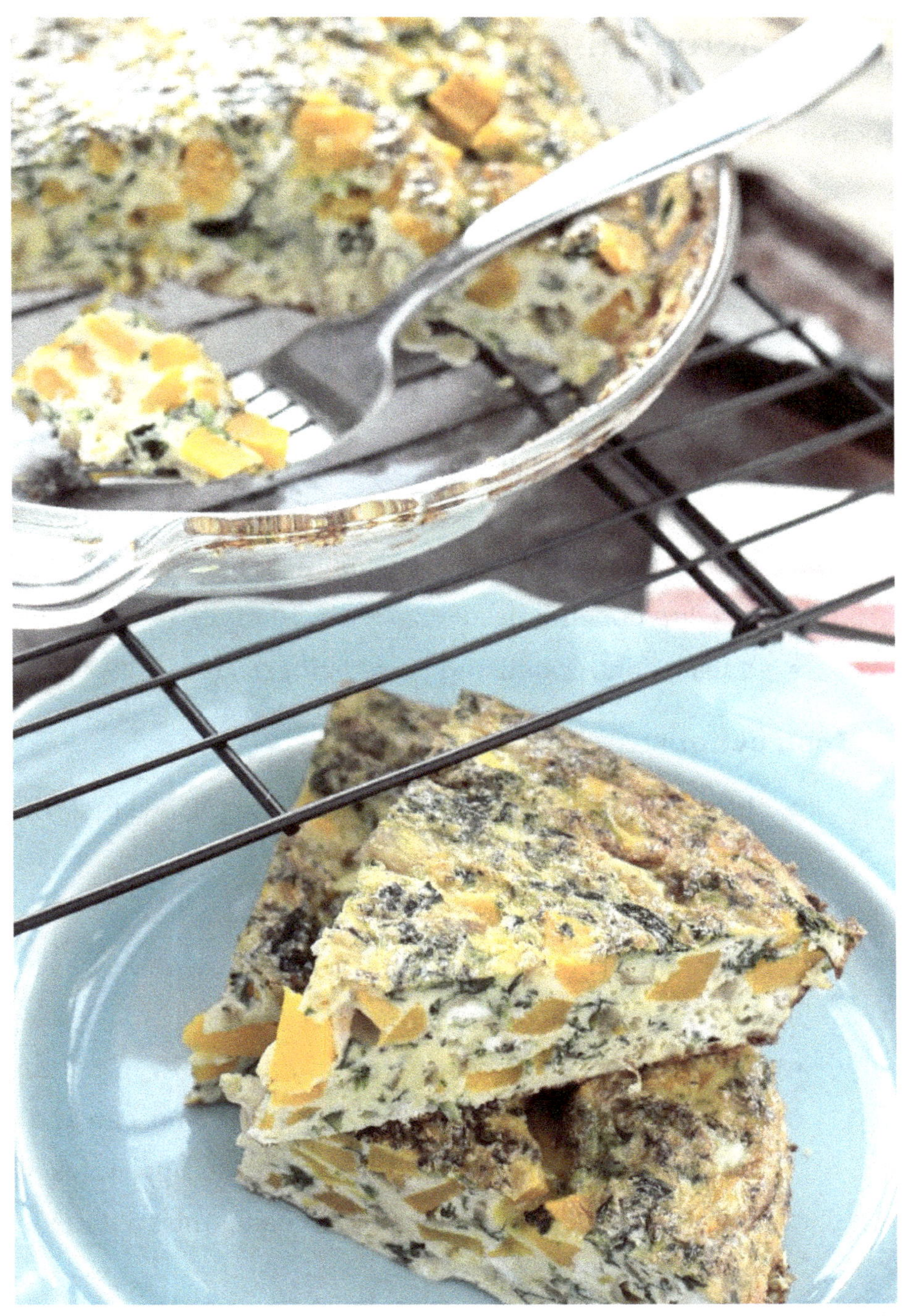

Sriracha-Ginger Chicken

Servings per Recipe: 3

Cooking Time: 25 minutes

Ingredients:

- ¼ cup fish sauce /62.5ML
- ¼ cup sriracha /62.5ML
- ½ cup light brown sugar /65G
- ½ cup rice vinegar /125ML
- 1 ½ pounds chicken breasts, pounded /675G
- 1/3 cup hot chili paste /83ML
- 2 teaspoons grated and peeled ginger /10G

Instructions:

1) Place all ingredients inside a Ziploc bag. Place in a fridge for some hours.
2) Preheat air fryer to 390° F or 199°C .
3) Place the grill pan in the air fryer.
4) Grill the chicken for 25 minutes.
5) Flip the chicken over every 10 minutes for even grilling.
6) Meanwhile, pour the marinade inside a saucepan and warmth over a medium flame before the sauce thickens.
7) Before serving the chicken, brush using the sriracha sauce.

Nutrition information:

- Calories per serving: 415
- Carbs: 5.4g
- Protein: 49.3g
- Fat: 21.8g

Sriracha-vinegar Marinated Chicken

Servings per Recipe: 4

Cooking Time: 40 minutes

Ingredients:

- ¼ cup Thai fish sauce /62.5ML
- ¼ cups sriracha sauce 62.5ML
- ½ cup rice vinegar /125ML
- 1 tablespoons sugar /15G
- 2 garlic cloves, minced
- 2 pounds chicken breasts
- Juice from 1 lime, freshly squeezed
- Salt and pepper to taste

Instructions:

1) Place all ingredients in a Ziploc bag except for the corn. Allow to marinate in the fridge for at least 2 hours.
2) Preheat the air fryer to 390° F or 199°C .
3) Place the grill pan in the air fryer.
4) Grill the chicken for 40 minutes, turn over the chicken to grill evenly.
5) Meanwhile, pour the marinade in a saucepan and place the saucepan over medium flame until it thickens.
6) Brush the chicken with the sauce. Serve with cucumbers if desired.

Nutrition information:

- Calories per serving: 427
- Carbs: 6.7g
- Protein: 49.1g
- Fat: 22.6g

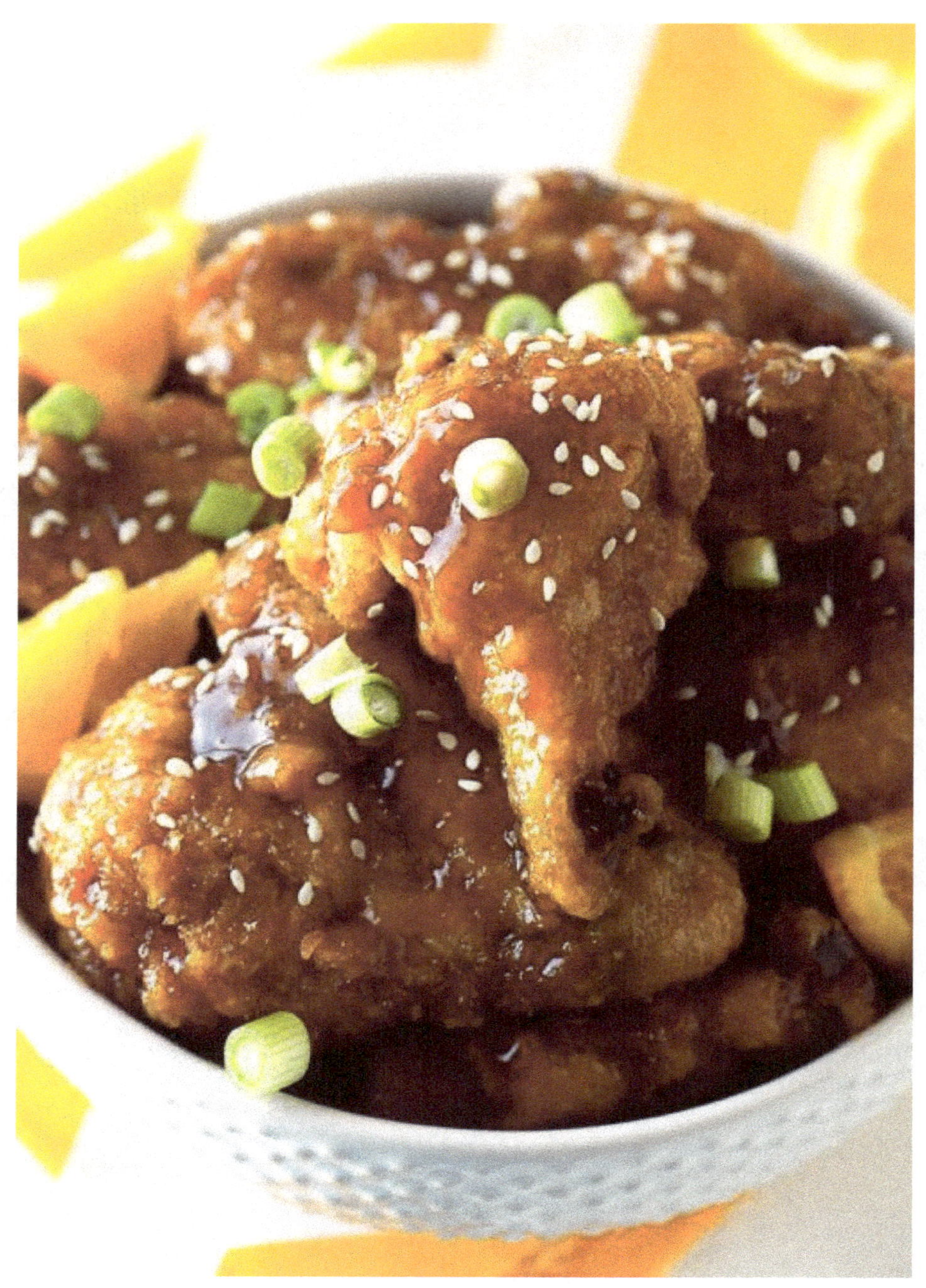

Sticky-Sweet Chicken BBQ

Servings per Recipe: 2

Cooking Time: 40 minutes

Ingredients:

- ½ cup balsamic vinegar /125ML
- ½ cup soy sauce /125ML
- 1-pound chicken drumsticks /450G
- 2 cloves of garlic, minced
- 2 green onion, sliced thinly
- 2 tablespoons sesame seeds /30G
- 3 tablespoons honey /45ML

Instructions:

1) Place the soy sauce, balsamic vinegar, honey, garlic, and chicken in a Ziploc bag, mix to combine. Place in the fridge for 30 minutes and allow to marinate.
2) Preheat air fryer to 330° F or 166°C .
3) Place the grill pan in the air fryer.
4) Place on the grill and cook for 30-40 minutes. Turnover the chicken every 10 minutes to grill evenly.
5) Meanwhile, Place the marinade in a saucepan. Simmer before the sauce thickens.

6) Once the chicken is cooked, brush with all the thickened marinade and garnish with sesame seeds and green onions.

Nutrition information:

- Calories per serving: 594
- Carbs: 43.7g
- Protein: 48.7g
- Fat: 24.9g

Sweet Lime 'n Chili Chicken Barbecue

Servings per Recipe: 2

Cooking Time: 40 minutes

Ingredients

- ¼ cup soy sauce /62.5ML
- 1 cup sweet chili sauce /250ML
- 1-pound chicken breasts /450G
- Juice from 2 limes, freshly squeezed

Instructions:

1) Combine all ingredients in a Ziploc bag and shake well. Allow to marinate for about 2 hours in the fridge.
2) Preheat mid-air fryer to 390° F or 199°C .
3) Place the grill pan in the air fryer.
4) Place chicken on the grill and cook for 40 to 50 minutes. Flip the chicken over every 10 minutes to cook evenly.
5) Meanwhile, Put the remaining marinade in a saucepan. Simmer before the sauce thickens.
6) Brush the cooked chicken with all the thickened marinade and serve.

Nutrition information:

- Calories per serving: 563
- Carbs: 39.2g

- Protein: 43.6g
- Fat: 25.7g

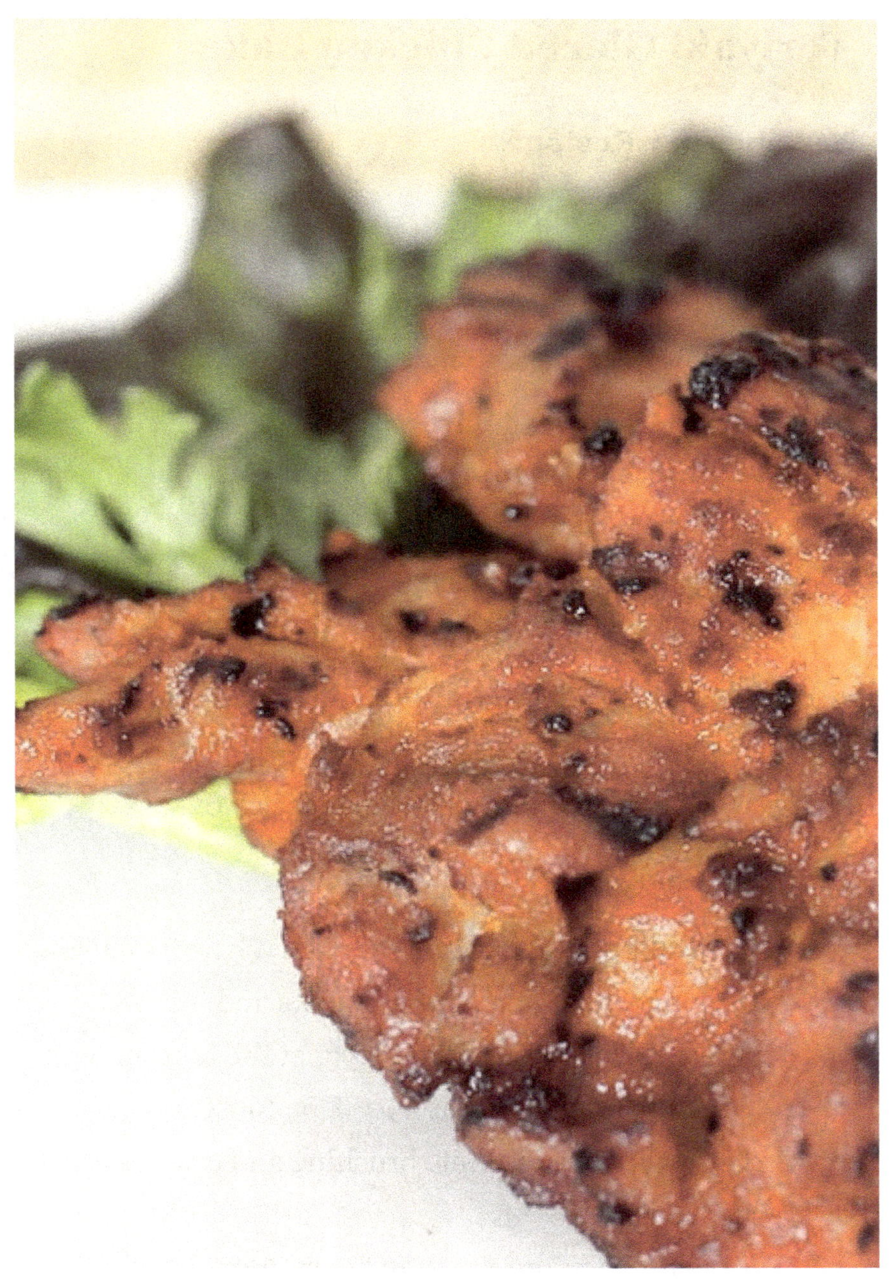

Teriyaki Glazed Chicken Bake

Servings per Recipe: 2

Cooking Time: 25 minutes

Ingredients:

- 2 tablespoons cider vinegar /30ML
- 4 skinless chicken thighs
- 1-1/2 teaspoons cornstarch /7.5G
- 1-1/2 teaspoons cold water /7.5ML
- 1/2 clove garlic, minced
- 1/4 cup white sugar /32.5G
- 1/4 cup soy sauce /62.5ML
- 1/4 teaspoon ground ginger /1.25G
- 1/8 teaspoon ground black pepper /0.625G

Instructions:

1) Grease the baking pan of the air fryer with oil using a cooking spray. Add all ingredients and mix well to coat. Spread chicken in a single layer at the bottom of the pan.
2) For 15 minutes, cook at 390° F or 199°C .
3) Turnover chicken while brushing and coating well with the sauce.
4) Cook for 15 minutes at 330° F or 166°C .
5) Serve and enjoy.

Nutrition Information:

- Calories per Serving: 267
- Carbs: 19.9g
- Protein: 24.7g
- Fat: 9.8g

Tomato, Cheese 'n Broccoli Quiche

Servings per Recipe: 2

Cooking Time: 24 minutes

Ingredients

- ½ cup Cheddar Cheese grated /65G
- ½ cup Whole Milk /125ML
- 1 Large Carrot, peeled and diced
- 1 Large Tomato, chopped
- 1 small Broccoli, cut into florets
- 1 Tsp Parsley /5G
- 1 Tsp Thyme /5G
- 2 Large Eggs
- 2 tbsp Feta Cheese /30G
- Salt & Pepper

Instructions:

1) Grease the baking pan of the air fryer with cooking spray.
2) Spread carrots, broccoli, and tomato in the baking pan.
3) For 10 minutes, cook at 330° F or 166°C .
4) Meanwhile, in a medium-sized bowl whisk eggs and milk well. Season generously with pepper and salt. Sprinkle parsley and thyme.

5) Remove the basket and add a little of the condiment. Sprinkle cheddar cheese. Pour egg mixture over vegetables and cheese.

6) Cook for another 12 minutes or until your preferred doneness.

7) Sprinkle feta cheese and allow it sit for two minutes.

8) Serve and enjoy.

Nutrition Information:

- Calories per Serving: 363
- Carbs: 23.7g
- Protein: 21.0g
- Fat: 20.4g

Tomato, Eggplant 'n Chicken Skewers

Servings per Recipe: 4

Cooking Time: 25 minutes

Ingredients:

- ¼ teaspoon cayenne /1.25G
- ¼ teaspoon ground cardamom /1.25G
- 1 ½ teaspoon ground turmeric /7.5G
- 1 can coconut milk /250ML
- 1 cup cherry tomatoes /130G
- 1 medium eggplant, cut into cubes
- 1 onion, cut into wedges
- 1-inch ginger, grated
- 2 pounds boneless chicken breasts, cut into cubes /900G
- 2 tablespoons fresh lime juice /30ML
- 2 tablespoons tomato paste /30ML
- 3 teaspoons lime zest /15G
- 4 cloves of garlic, minced
- Salt and pepper to taste

Instructions:

1) Place garlic, ginger, coconut milk, lime zest, lime juice, tomato paste, salt, pepper, turmeric, red pepper cayenne, cardamom, and chicken breasts in a bowl. Allow to marinate in the fridge for at least a couple of hours.

2) Preheat mid-air fryer to 390° F or 199°C .

3) Place the grill pan in a mid-air fryer.

4) Skewer the chicken cubes with eggplant, onion, and cherry tomatoes on bamboo skewers.

5) Place around the grill pan and cook for 25 minutes, turn over the chicken every 5 minutes while cooking.

Nutrition information:

- Calories per serving: 485
- Carbs:19.7 g
- Protein: 55.2g
- Fat: 20.6g

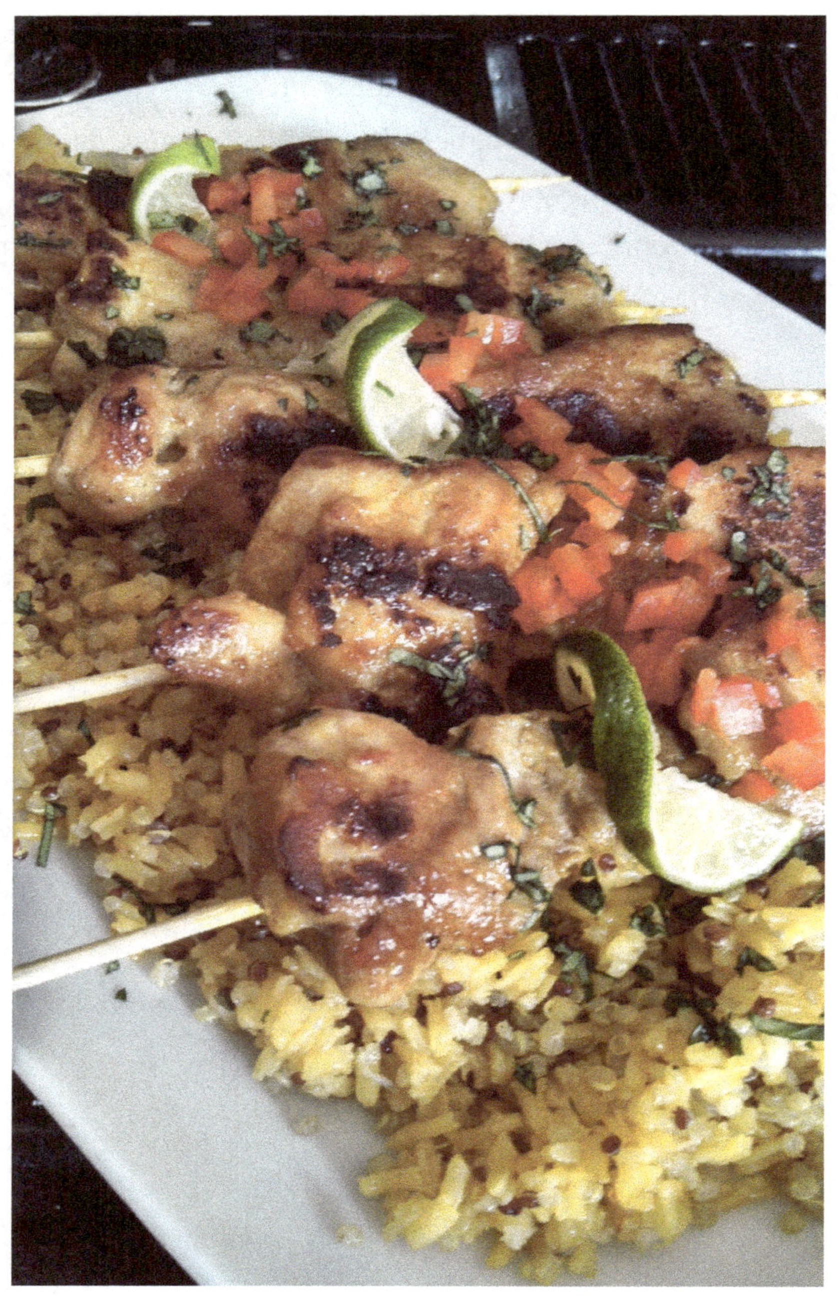

Turmeric and Lemongrass Chicken Roast

Servings per Recipe: 6

Cooking Time: 40 minutes

Ingredients:

- 1 teaspoon turmeric /5G
- 2 lemongrass stalks
- 2 tablespoons fish sauce /30ML
- 3 cloves of garlic, minced
- 3 pounds whole chicken /1150G
- 3 shallots, chopped
- Salt and pepper to taste

Instructions:

1) Place all ingredients in the Ziploc bag and marinate for at least 120 minutes in the fridge.
2) Preheat the air fryer to 390 F or 199°C .
3) Place the grill pan in mid-air fryer.
4) Grill the chicken for 40 minutes and flip over every 10 minutes during grilling.

Nutrition information:

- Calories per serving: 495
- Carbs: 49.1g

- Protein: 38.5g;
- Fat: 16.1g

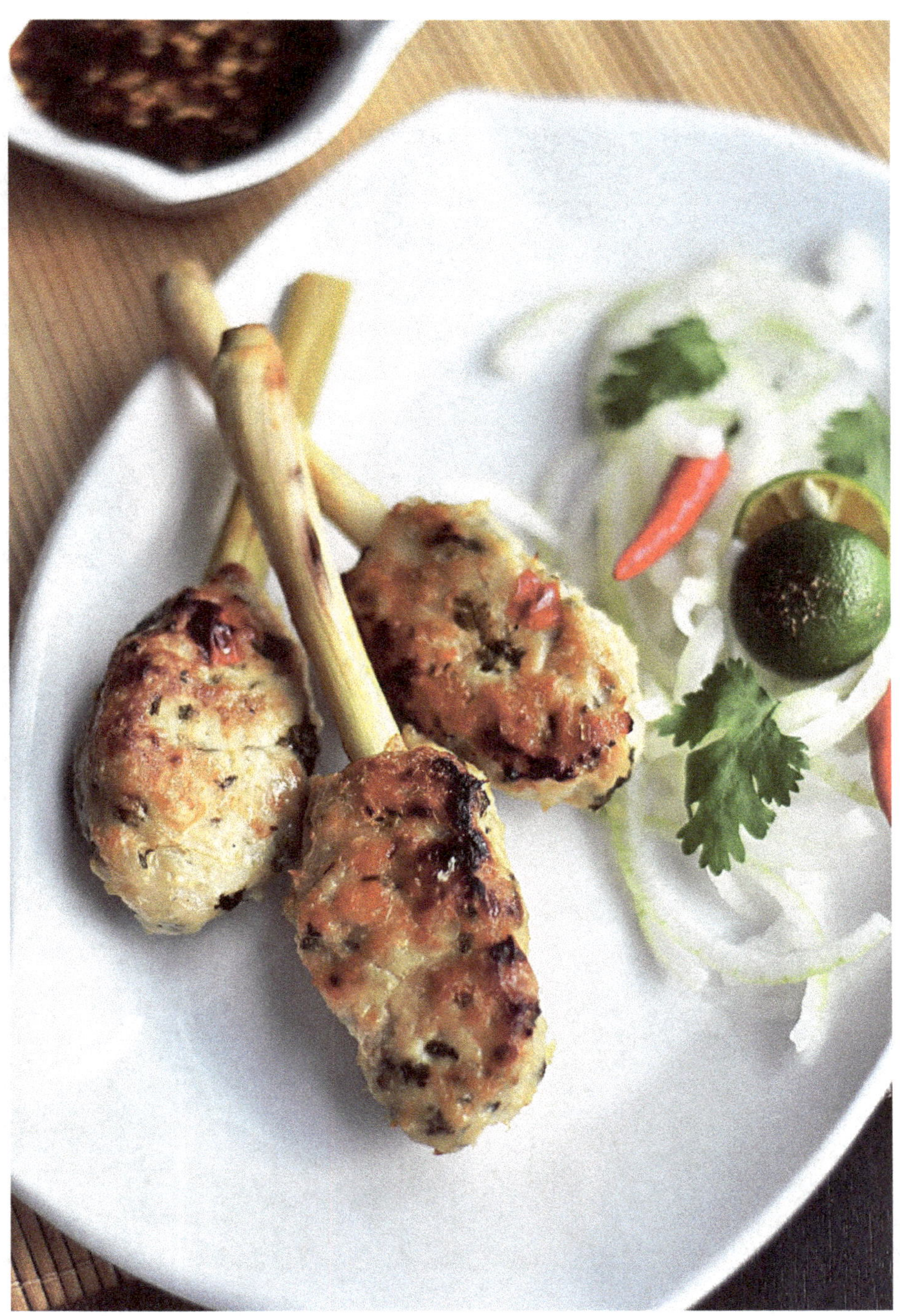

DESSERT

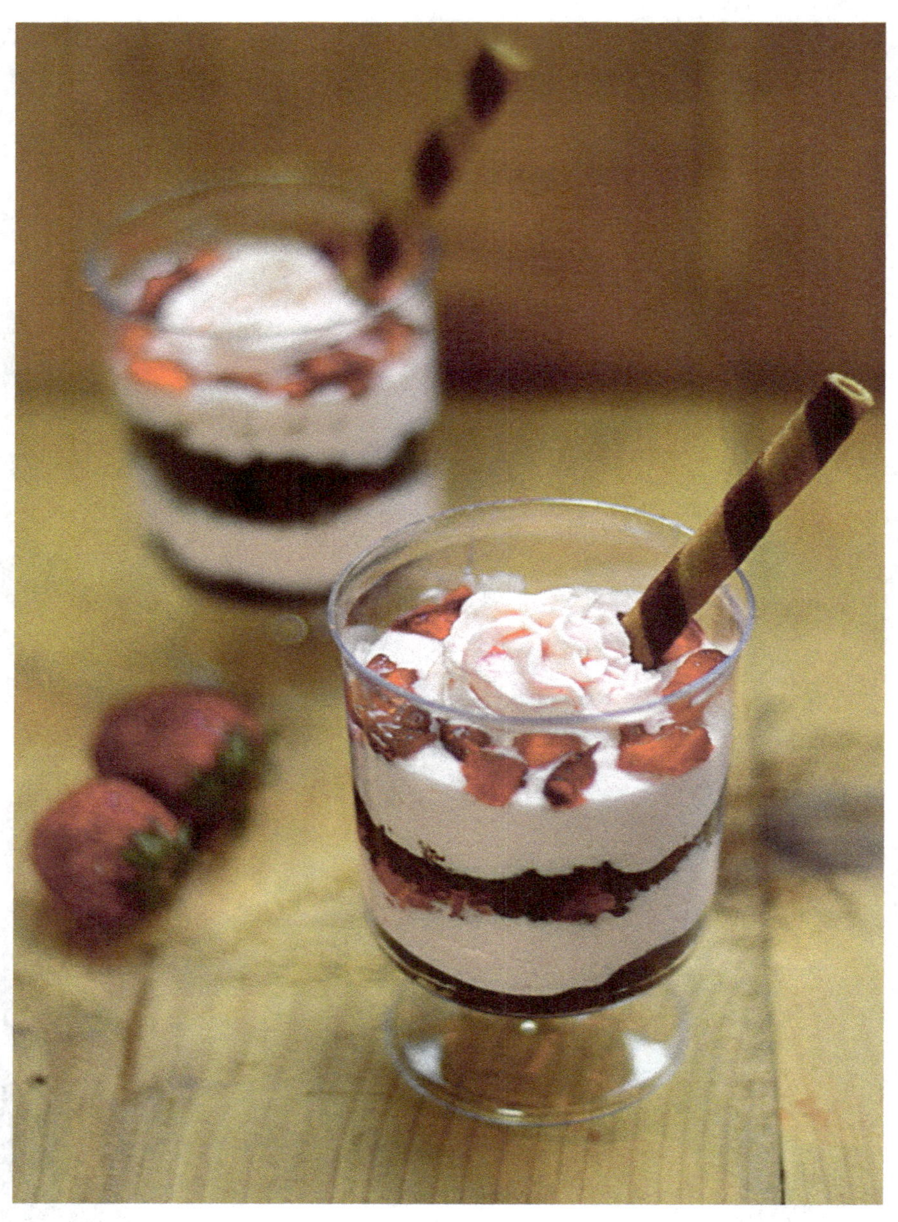

Apple Pie in Air Fryer

Servings per Recipe: 4

Cooking Time: 35 minutes

Ingredients:

- ½ teaspoon vanilla flavoring /2.5ML
- 1 beaten egg
- 1 large apple, chopped
- 1 Pillsbury Refrigerator pie crust
- 1 tablespoon butter /15G
- 1 tablespoon ground cinnamon /15G
- 1 tablespoon raw sugar /15G
- 2 tablespoon sugar /15G
- 2 teaspoons fresh lemon juice /10ML
- Baking spray

Instructions:

1) Using a cooking spray grease lightly the baking pan of an air fryer. Spread pie crust in the pan evenly.
2) Mix vanilla, sugar, cinnamon, lemon juice, and apples in a bowl. Pour this mixture on top of the pie crust. Add apples with butter slice on top too.
3) Cover using the remaining pie crust. Pierce the top of the pie with a knife.

4) Spread beaten eggs on top of the crust and sprinkle with sugar.
5) Cover with foil.
6) Cook at 390° F or 199°C for 25 minutes.
7) Remove foil and cook for an additional 10 minutes at 330° F or 166°C or until tops are brown.
8) Serve and enjoy.

Nutrition Information:

- Calories per Serving: 372
- Carbs: 44.7g
- Protein: 4.2g
- Fat: 19.6g

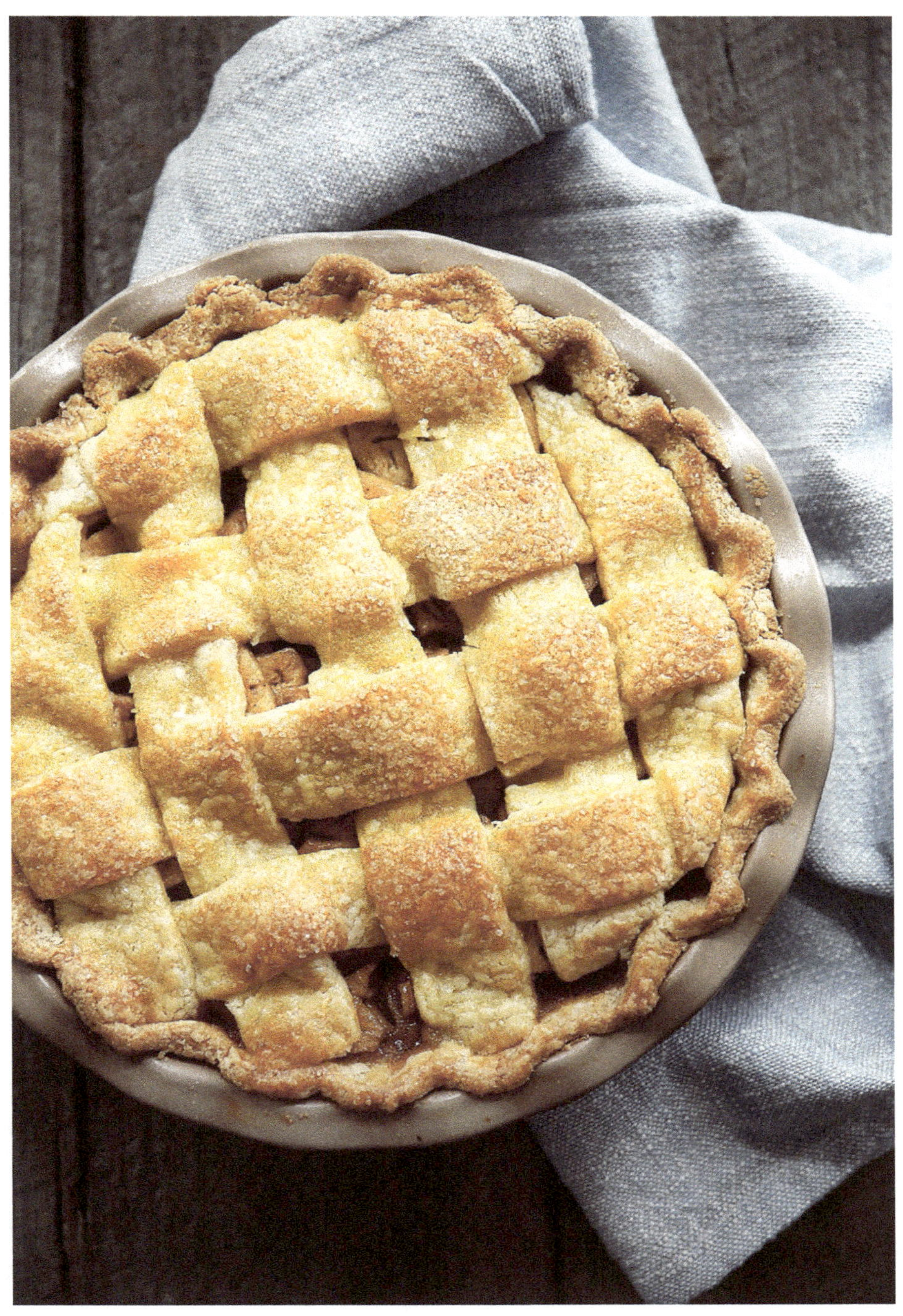

Apple-Toffee Upside-Down Cake

Serves: 9

Cooking Time: 30 Minutes

Ingredients

- ¼ cup almond butter /32.5G
- ¼ cup sunflower oil /62.5ML
- ½ cup walnuts, chopped /65G
- ¾ cup + 3 tablespoon coconut sugar /138G
- ¾ cup water /188ML
- 1 ½ teaspoon mixed spice /7.5G
- 1 cup plain flour /130G
- 1 lemon, zest
- 1 teaspoon baking soda /5G
- 1 teaspoon vinegar /5ML
- 3 baking apples, cored and sliced

Instructions:

1) Preheat air fryer to 390° F or 199°C .
2) Melt the almond butter and 3 tablespoons of sugar in a pan. Pour the mixture into the baking dish. Arrange the slices of apples on top. Set aside.
3) Add flour, ¾ cup sugar, and baking soda. Add the mixed spice.

4) Mix the oil, water, vinegar, and lemon zest. Add chopped walnuts and stir.

5) Combine both wet ingredients and dry ingredients. Mix well until well combined.

6) Place apple slices in the pan.

7) Bake for 30 minutes or place a toothpick in the middle of the pie if it comes out clean then the pie is cooked.

Nutrition information:

- Calories per serving: 335
- Carbohydrates: 39.6g
- Protein: 3.8g
- Fat: 17.9g

Banana-Choco Brownies

Serves: 12

Cooking Time: 30 Minutes

Ingredients:

- 2 cups almond flour /260G
- 2 teaspoons baking powder /10G
- ½ teaspoon baking powder /2.5G
- ½ teaspoon baking soda /2.5G
- ½ teaspoon salt /2.5G
- 1 over-ripe banana
- 3 large eggs
- ½ teaspoon stevia powder /2.5G
- ¼ cup coconut oil /62.5ML
- 1 tablespoon vinegar /15ML
- 1/3 cup almond flour /43G
- 1/3 cup hot chocolate mix /43G

Instructions:

1) Preheat the air fryer for 5 minutes.
2) Blend all ingredients.
3) Pour the mixture into a baking dish.
4) Place in the air fryer basket and cook for 30 minutes at 350° F or 177°C or if a toothpick inserted in the middle comes out clean.

Nutrition information:

- Calories per serving: 75
- Carbohydrates: 2.1g
- Protein: 1.7g
- Fat: 6.6g

Blueberry & Lemon Cake

Servings per Recipe: 4

Cooking Time: 17 minutes

Ingredients:

- 2 eggs
- 1 cup blueberries /130G
- zest from 1 lemon
- juice from 1 lemon
- 1 tsp. vanilla /5ML
- brown sugar for topping (somewhat sprinkling together with each muffin-less than a teaspoon)
- 2 1/2 cups self-rising flour /325G
- 1/2 cup Monk Fruit (or use your preferred sugar) /65G
- 1/2 cup cream /125ML
- 1/4 cup avocado oil (any light cooking oil) /62.5ML

Instructions:

1) Place all ingredients in a mixing bowl and mix. Add the dry ingredients and mix well.
2) Grease baking pan lightly with oil using cooking spray. Pour the batter in.
3) Cook at 330° F or 166°C for 12 minutes.
4) Let it stay at home air fryer for 5 minutes.
5) Serve, eat and enjoy.

Nutrition Information:

- Calories per Serving: 589
- Carbs: 76.7g
- Protein: 13.5g
- Fat: 25.3g

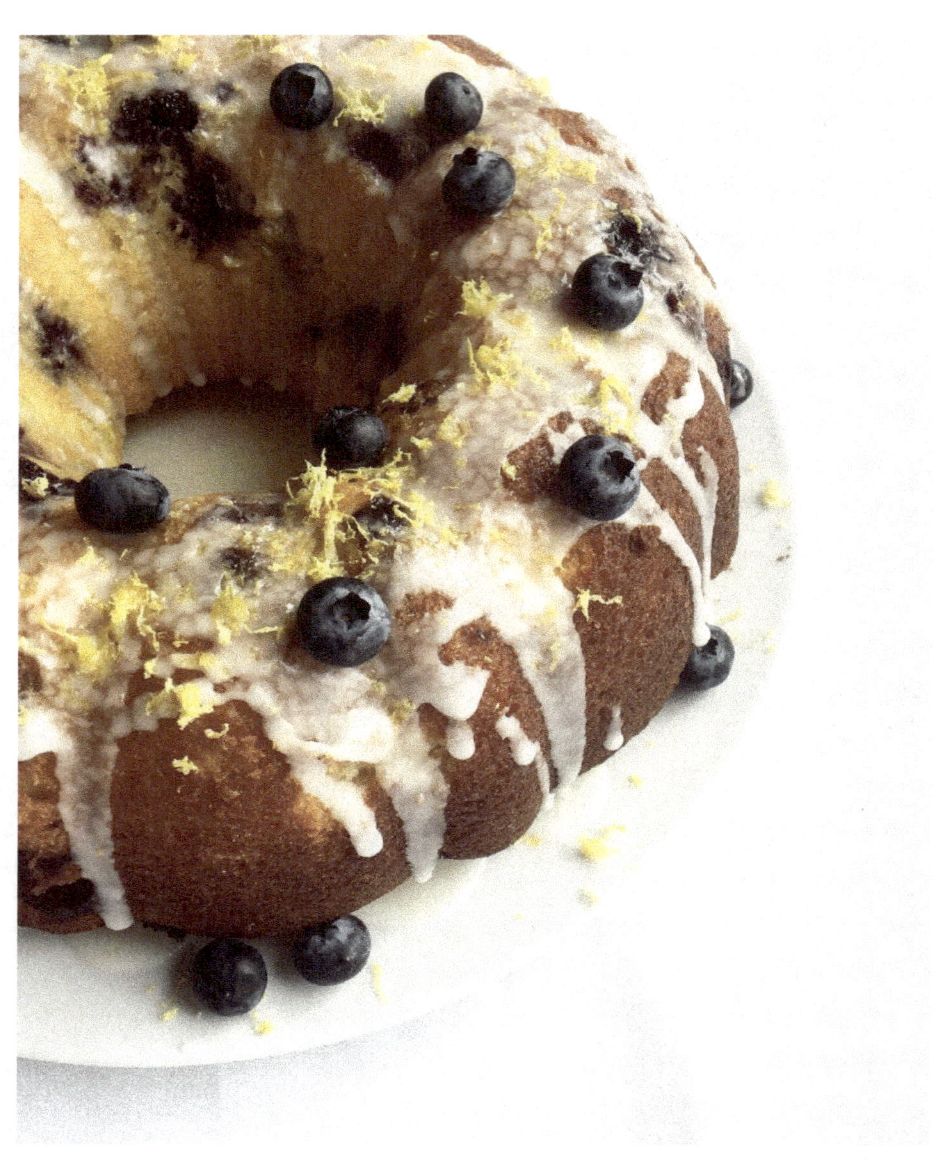

Bread Pudding with Cranberry

Servings per Recipe: 4

Cooking Time: 45 minutes

Ingredients:

- 1-1/2 cups milk /375ML
- 2-1/2 eggs
- 1/2 cup cranberries1 teaspoon butter /70G
- 1/4 cup and two tablespoons white sugar /62.5G
- 1/4 cup golden raisins /32.5G
- 1/8 teaspoon ground cinnamon /0.625G
- 3/4 cup heavy whipping cream /188ML
- 3/4 teaspoon lemon zest /3.75G
- 3/4 teaspoon kosher salt /3.75G
- 3/4 French baguettes, cut into 2-inch slices
- 3/8 vanilla bean, split and seeds scraped away

Instructions:

1) Grease baking pan with oil. Spread baguette slices, cranberries, and raisins in the pan.
2) Blend vanilla bean, cinnamon, salt, lemon zest, eggs, sugar, and cream. Pour this mixture over baguette slices. Let it soak for an hour.
3) Cover pan with foil.
4) Cook for 35 minutes at 330° F or 166°C .

5) Let it sit for 10 minutes.

6) Serve and enjoy

Nutrition Information:

- Calories per Serving: 581
- Carbs: 76.1g
- Protein: 15.8g
- Fat: 23.7g

Cherries 'n Almond Flour Bars

Serves: 12

Cooking Time: 35 minutes

Ingredients

- ¼ cup water /62.5ML
- ½ cup butter softened /65G
- ½ teaspoon salt / 2.5G
- ½ teaspoon vanilla /2.5G
- 1 ½ cups almond flour /195G
- 1 cup erythritol /130G
- 1 cup fresh cherries, pitted /130G
- 1 tablespoon xanthan gum /15G
- 2 eggs

Instructions:

1) Add the first 6 ingredients to a mixing bowl, mix well to form a dough.
2) Add the dough to the baking pan.
3) Place in the air fryer and bake for 10 minutes at 375° F or 191°C .
4) Meanwhile, mix the cherries, water, and xanthan gum in a bowl.
5) Take the dough out and pour on the cherry mixture.
6) Return the baking pan to the mid-air fryer and cook again for 25 minutes at 375° F or 191°C .

Nutrition information:

- Calories per serving: 99
- Carbohydrates: 2.1g
- Protein: 1.8g
- Fat: 9.3g

Cherry-Choco Bars

Serves: 8

Cooking Time: 15

Ingredients:

- ¼ teaspoon salt /1.25G
- ½ cup almonds, sliced /65G
- ½ cup chia seeds /65G
- ½ cup chocolate brown, chopped /65G
- ½ cup dried cherries, chopped /65G
- ½ cup prunes, pureed /65G
- ½ cup quinoa, cooked /65G
- ¾ cup almond butter /98G
- 1/3 cup honey /83ML
- 2 cups old-fashioned oats /260G
- 2 tablespoon coconut oil /30ML

Instructions:

1) Preheat mid-air fryer to 375° F or 191°C .
2) Add the oats, quinoa, chia seeds, almond, cherries, and chocolate to a mixing bowl, mix well to combine.
3) Heat the almond butter, honey, and coconut oil.
4) Pour the butter mixture into the dry mixture. Add salt and prunes.
5) Mix until well combined.

6) Pour the mixture into the baking dish.

7) Cook for 15 minutes.

8) Let it cool for an hour before slicing it into bars.

Nutrition information:

- Calories per serving: 321

- Carbohydrates: 35g

- Protein: 7g

- Fat: 17g

Chocolate Chip inside a Mug

Serves: 6

Cooking Time: 20 Minutes

Ingredients:

- ¼ cup walnuts, shelled and chopped /32.5G
- ½ cup butter, unsalted /65G
- ½ cup chocolate bars chips /65G
- ½ cup erythritol /65G
- ½ teaspoon baking soda /2.5G
- ½ teaspoon salt /2.5G
- 1 tablespoon vanilla extract /15ML
- 2 ½ cups almond flour /325G
- 2 large eggs, beaten

Instructions%

1) Preheat the air fryer for 5 minutes.
2) Combine all ingredients in the mixing bowl. Mix well.
3) Place in greased pans.
4) Bake in mid-air fryer for 20 minutes at 375° F or 191°C .

Nutrition information:

1) Calories per serving: 234
2) Carbohydrates: 4.9g
3) Protein: 2.3g

4) Fat: 22.8g

Choco-Peanut Mug Cake

Serves: 1

Cooking Time: 20 minutes

Ingredients

- ¼ teaspoon baking powder /1.25G
- ½ teaspoon vanilla flavor /2.5ML
- 1 egg
- 1 tablespoon heavy cream /15ML
- 1 tablespoon peanut butter /15G
- 1 teaspoon butter, softened /5G
- 2 tablespoon erythritol /30G
- 2 tablespoons cocoa powder, unsweetened /30G

Instructions:

1) Preheat mid-air fryer for 5 minutes.
2) Combine all ingredients in a mixing bowl.
3) Pour into a greased pan.
4) Place in mid-air fryer basket and cook for 20 minutes at 400° F or 205°C or if a toothpick comes clean when inserted in the middle of the pie.

Nutrition information:

- Calories per serving: 293
- Carbohydrates:8.5g

- Protein: 12.4g
- Fat: 23.3g

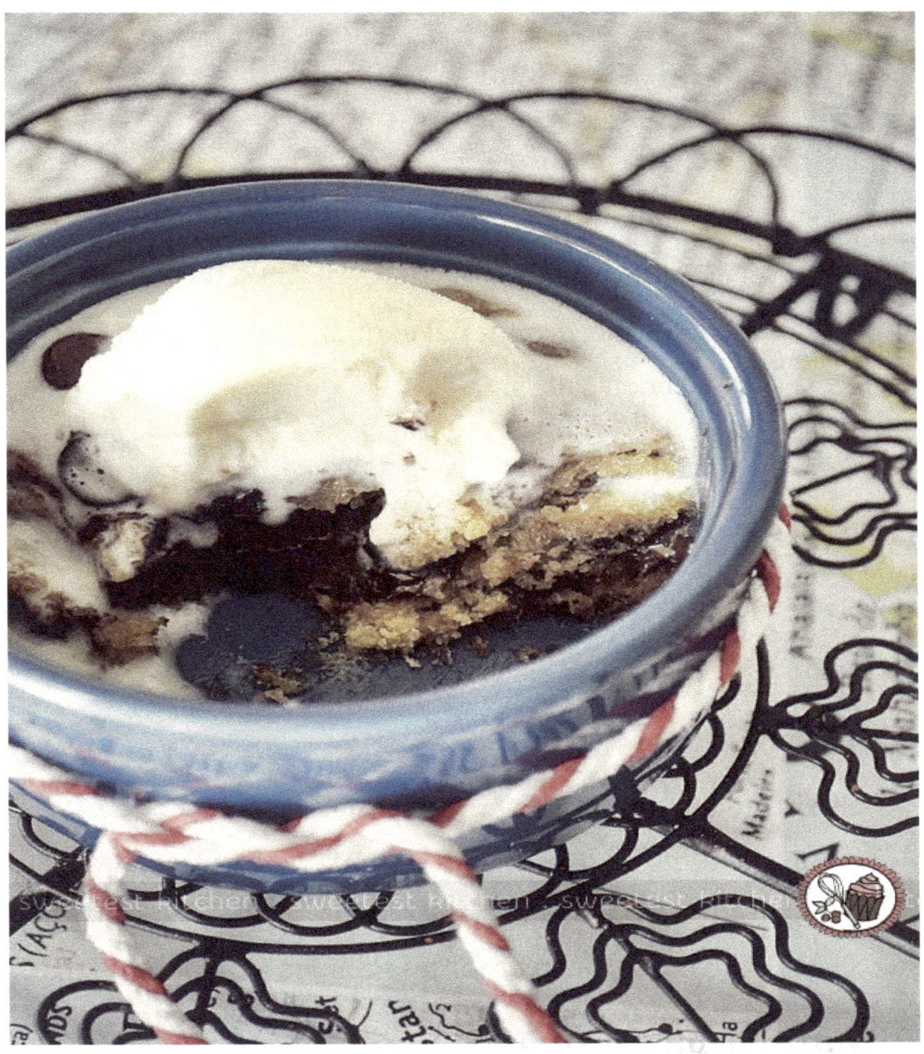

Coco-Lime Bars

Serves: 3

Cooking Time: 20 minutes

Ingredients:

- ¼ cup almond flour /32.5G
- ¼ cup coconut oil /62.5ML
- ¼ cup dried coconut flakes/32.5G
- ¼ teaspoon salt /1.25G
- ½ cup lime juice /125ML
- ¾ cup coconut flour /98G
- 1 ¼ cup erythritol powder /162.5G
- 1 tablespoon lime zest /15G
- 4 eggs

Instructions:

1) Preheat mid-air fryer for 5 minutes.
2) Combine all ingredients in a mixing bowl. Mix well.
3) Pour ingredients into the pan.
4) Bake in the air fryer for 20 minutes at 375° F or 191°C .

Nutrition information:

- Calories per serving: 506
- Carbohydrates: 21.9g
- Protein: 19.3g

- Fat: 37.9g

Coconut 'n Almond Fat Bombs

Serves: 12

Cooking Time: 15 minutes

Ingredients

- ¼ cup almond flour /32.5G
- ½ cup shredded coconut /65G
- 1 tablespoon coconut oil /15ML
- 1 tablespoon vanilla extract /15ML
- 2 tablespoons liquid stevia /30ML
- 3 egg whites

Instructions:

1) Preheat the air fryer for 5 minutes.
2) Combine all ingredients inside a mixing bowl. Mix well.
3) Form small balls of patties using your hands.
4) Place in mid-air fryer basket and cook for 15 minutes at 400° F or 205°C .

Nutrition information:

- Calories per serving: 23
- Carbohydrates: 0.7g
- Protein: 1.1g
- Fat: 1.8g

Coconutty Lemon Bars

Serves: 12

Cooking Time: 25 minutes

Ingredients:

- ¼ cup cashew /32.5G
- ¼ cup fresh lemon juice, freshly squeezed /62.5ML
- ¾ cup coconut milk /188ML
- ¾ cup erythritol /98G
- 1 cup desiccated coconut /130G
- 1 teaspoon baking powder /5G
- 2 eggs, beaten
- 2 tablespoons coconut oil /30ML
- A dash of salt

Instructions

1) Preheat the air fryer for 5 minutes.
2) Combine all ingredients and mix well.
3) Use a hand mixer to blend everything.
4) Pour into a baking dish.
5) Bake for 25 minutes at 350° F or 177°C or until a toothpick inserted in middle comes clean.

Nutrition information:

- Calories per serving: 118

- Carbohydrates: 3.9g
- Protein: 2.6g
- Fat:10.2g

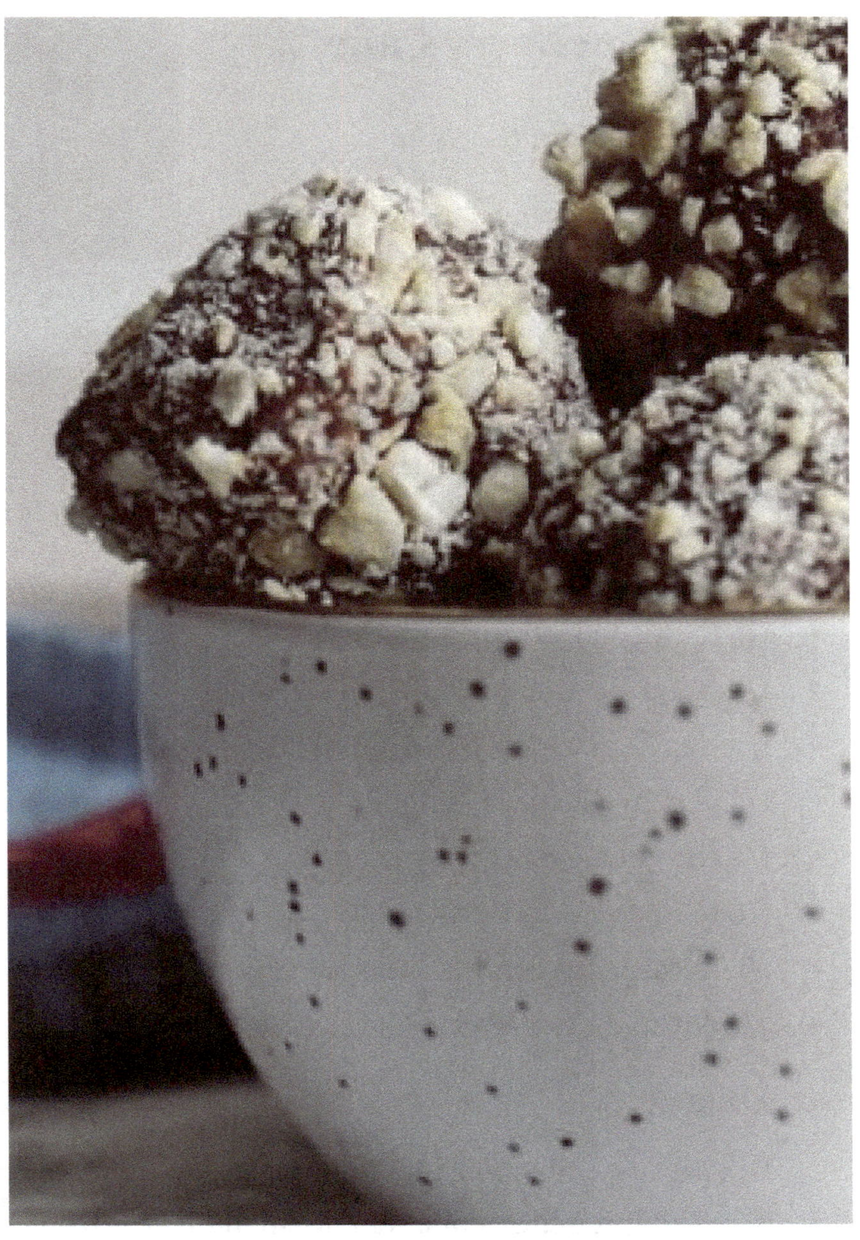

Coffee 'n Blueberry Cake

Servings per Recipe: 6

Cooking Time: 35 minutes

Ingredients:

- 1 cup white sugar /130G
- 1 egg
- 1/2 cup butter, softened /65G
- 1/2 cup fresh or frozen blueberries /65G
- 1/2 cup sour cream /125ML
- 1/2 teaspoon baking powder /2.5G
- 1/2 teaspoon ground cinnamon /2.5G
- 1/2 teaspoon vanilla flavoring /2.5G
- 1/4 cup brown sugar /32.5G
- 1/4 cup chopped pecans /32.5G
- 1/8 teaspoon salt /0.625G
- 1-1/2 teaspoons confectioners' sugar for dusting /7.5G
- 3/4 cup and 1 tablespoon all-purpose flour /112.5G

Instructions:

1) Mix pecans, cinnamon, and brown sugar.
2) Blend all wet ingredients. Add dry ingredients except confectioner's sugar and blueberries. Blend well until smooth and creamy.
3) Grease baking pan with oil.

4) Pour half of the batter into the pan. Sprinkle ½ of pecan mixture on top. Pour the remaining batter. And top with the remaining pecan mixture.
5) Cover pan with foil.
6) Cook for 35 minutes at 330° F or 166°C .
7) Serve with a dusting of confectioner's sugar and enjoy.

Nutrition Information:

- Calories per Serving: 471
- Carbs: 59.5g
- Protein: 4.1g
- Fat: 24.0g

Coffee Flavored Cookie Dough

Serves: 12

Cooking Time: 20 Minutes

Ingredients:

- ¼ cup butter /32.5G
- ¼ teaspoon xanthan gum /1.25G
- ½ teaspoon coffee espresso powder /2.5G
- ½ teaspoon stevia powder /2.5G
- ¾ cup almond flour /98G
- 1 egg
- 1 teaspoon vanilla /5G
- 1/3 cup sesame seeds /43G
- 2 tablespoons cocoa powder /30G
- 2 tablespoons cream cheese, softened /30G

Instructions:

1) Preheat the air fryer for 5 minutes.
2) Combine all ingredients inside a mixing bowl.
3) Press right into a baking dish that can fit in the air fryer.
4) Place in mid-air fryer basket and cook for 20 minutes at 400° F or 205°C or if a toothpick inserted inside come out clean.

Nutrition information:

- Calories per serving: 88
- Carbohydrates: 1.3g
- Protein: 1.9g
- Fat: 8.3g

Coffee Flavored Doughnuts

Serves: 6

Cooking Time: 6 minutes

Ingredients:

- ¼ cup coconut sugar /32.5G
- ¼ cup coffee /32.5G
- ½ teaspoon salt /2.5G
- 1 cup white all-purpose flour /130G
- 1 tablespoon sunflower oil /15ML
- 1 teaspoon baking powder /5G
- 2 tablespoon aquafaba /30ML

Instructions:

1) Mix the dry ingredients flour, sugar, salt, and baking powder.
2) Mix the aquafaba, sunflower oil, and coffee.
3) Mix to make a dough.
4) Allow the dough to sit in the fridge.
5) Preheat air fryer to 400° F or 205°C .
6) Knead the dough and form doughnuts.
7) Place in a single layer in the air fryer and cook for 6 minutes.
8) Avoid shaking the pan to keep the donut in shape.

Nutrition information:

- Calories per serving: 113
- Carbohydrates: 20.45g
- Protein: 2.16g
- Fat:2.54g

Crisped 'n Chewy Chonut Holes

Serves: 6

Cooking Time: 10 minutes

Ingredients:

- ¼ cup almond milk /62.5ML
- ¼ cup coconut sugar /32.5G
- ¼ teaspoon cinnamon /1.25G
- ½ teaspoon salt /2.5G
- 1 cup white all-purpose flour /130G
- 1 tablespoon coconut oil, melted /15ML
- 1 teaspoon baking powder /5G
- 2 tablespoon aquafaba or liquid from canned chickpeas /30ML

Instructions:

1) Mix the flour, sugar, and baking powder in a bowl. Add the salt and cinnamon and mix well.
2) Mix the coconut oil, aquafaba, and almond milk in another bowl.
3) Gently pour the dry ingredients on the wet ingredients. Mix until well combined.
4) Place the dough inside a refrigerator to rest for about an hour.
5) Preheat mid-air fryer to 370° F or 191°C .

6) Make small balls with the dough and set them inside the air fryer and cook for 10 minutes. Do not shake the air fryer.

7) Once cooked, sprinkle with sugar and cinnamon.

8) Serve with your breakfast coffee.

Nutrition information:

- Calories per serving: 120
- Carbohydrates: 21.62g
- Protein: 2.31g
- Fat:2.76g

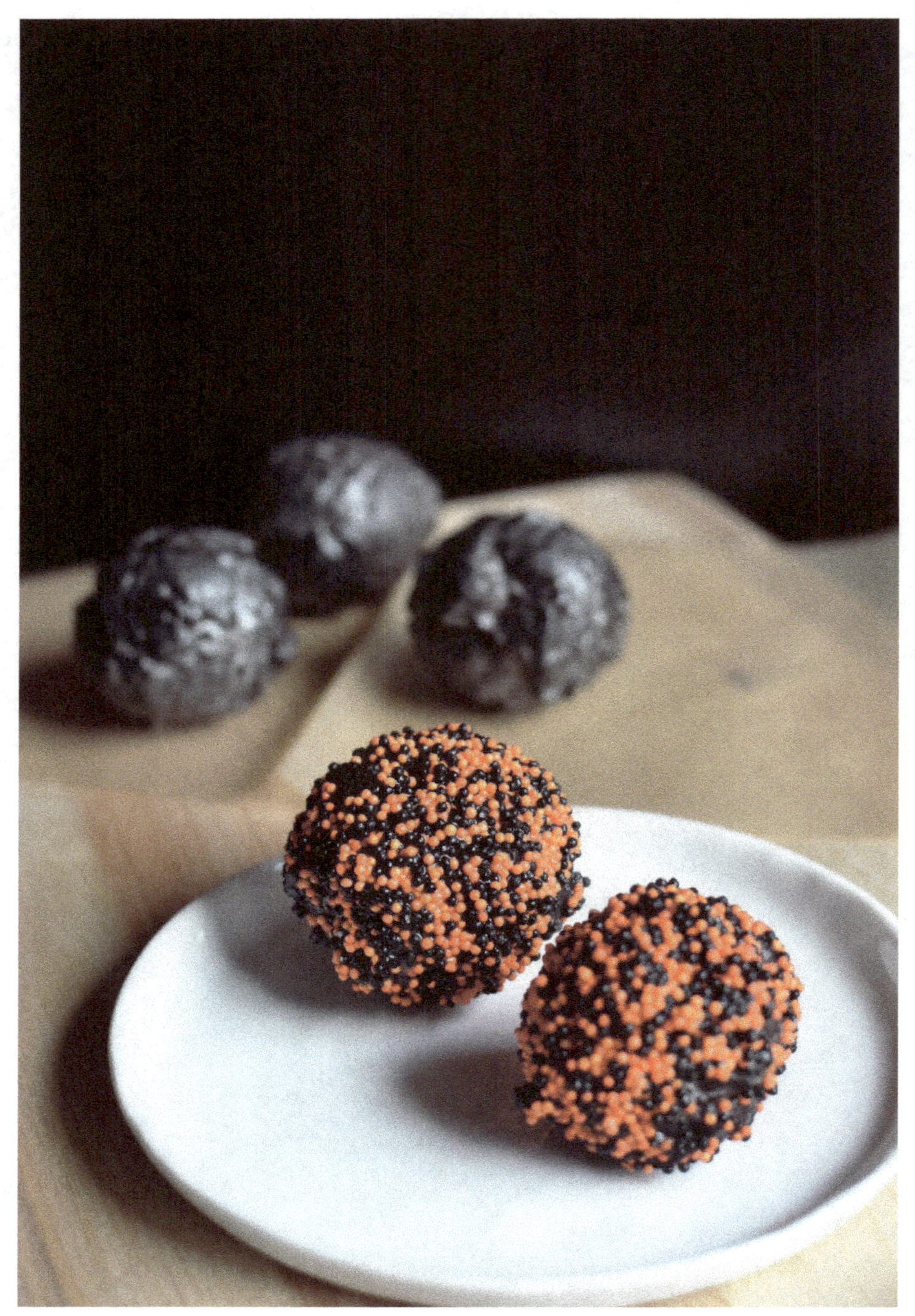

Crispy Good Peaches

Servings per Recipe: 4

Cooking Time: 30 minutes

Ingredients:

- 1 teaspoon cinnamon /5G
- 1 teaspoon sugar, white /5G
- 1/3 cup oats, dry rolled /43G
- 1/4 cup Flour, white /32.5G
- 2 tablespoon Flour, white /30G
- 3 tablespoon butter, unsalted /45G
- 3 tablespoon sugar /45G
- 3 tablespoon pecans, chopped /45G
- 4 cup sliced peaches, frozen /520G

Instructions:

1) Grease baking pan of air fryer with cooking spray. Mix in a tsp cinnamon, 2 tbsp flour, 3 tbsp sugar, and peaches.
2) Cook for 20 minutes at 300° F or 149°C .
3) Mix the rest of the ingredients in the bowl. Pour over peaches.
4) Cook for 10 minutes at 330° F or 166°C .
5) Serve and enjoy.

Nutrition Information:

- Calories per Serving: 435
- Carbs: 74.1g
- Protein: 4.3g
- Fat: 13.4g

Easy Baked Chocolate Mug Cake

Serves: 3

Cooking Time: 15

Ingredients:

- ½ cup cocoa powder /65G
- ½ cup stevia powder /65G
- 1 cup coconut cream /250ML
- 1 package cream cheese, room temperature
- 1 tablespoon vanilla flavoring /15ML
- 4 tablespoons butter /60ML

Instructions:

1) Preheat the air fryer for 5 minutes.
2) Combine all ingredients. Mix well.
3) Use a hand mixer to mix everything until fluffy.
4) Pour into greased pans.
5) Place the pan in the fryer basket.
6) Bake for 15 minutes at 350° F or 177°C .
7) Place inside the fridge to set before serving.

Nutrition information:

- Calories per serving: 744
- Carbohydrates:15.3 g
- Protein: 13.9g

- Fat: 69.7g

Hot Coconut 'n Cocoa Buns

Serves: 8

Preparation Time: 8 minutes

Cooking Time: 15

Ingredients:

- ¼ cup cacao nibs /32.5G
- 1 cup coconut milk /250ML
- 1/3 cup coconut flour /43G
- 3 tablespoons cacao powder /45G
- 4 eggs, beaten

Instructions:

1) Preheat the air fryer for 5 minutes.
2) Combine all ingredients inside a mixing bowl.
3) Form buns with your hands and place in the baking dish.
4) Bake for 15 minutes for 375° F or 191°C .
5) Leave the buns in the air fryer until it cools completely.

Nutrition information:

- Calories per serving: 161
- Carbohydrates: 4g
- Protein: 5.7g
- Fat: 13.6g

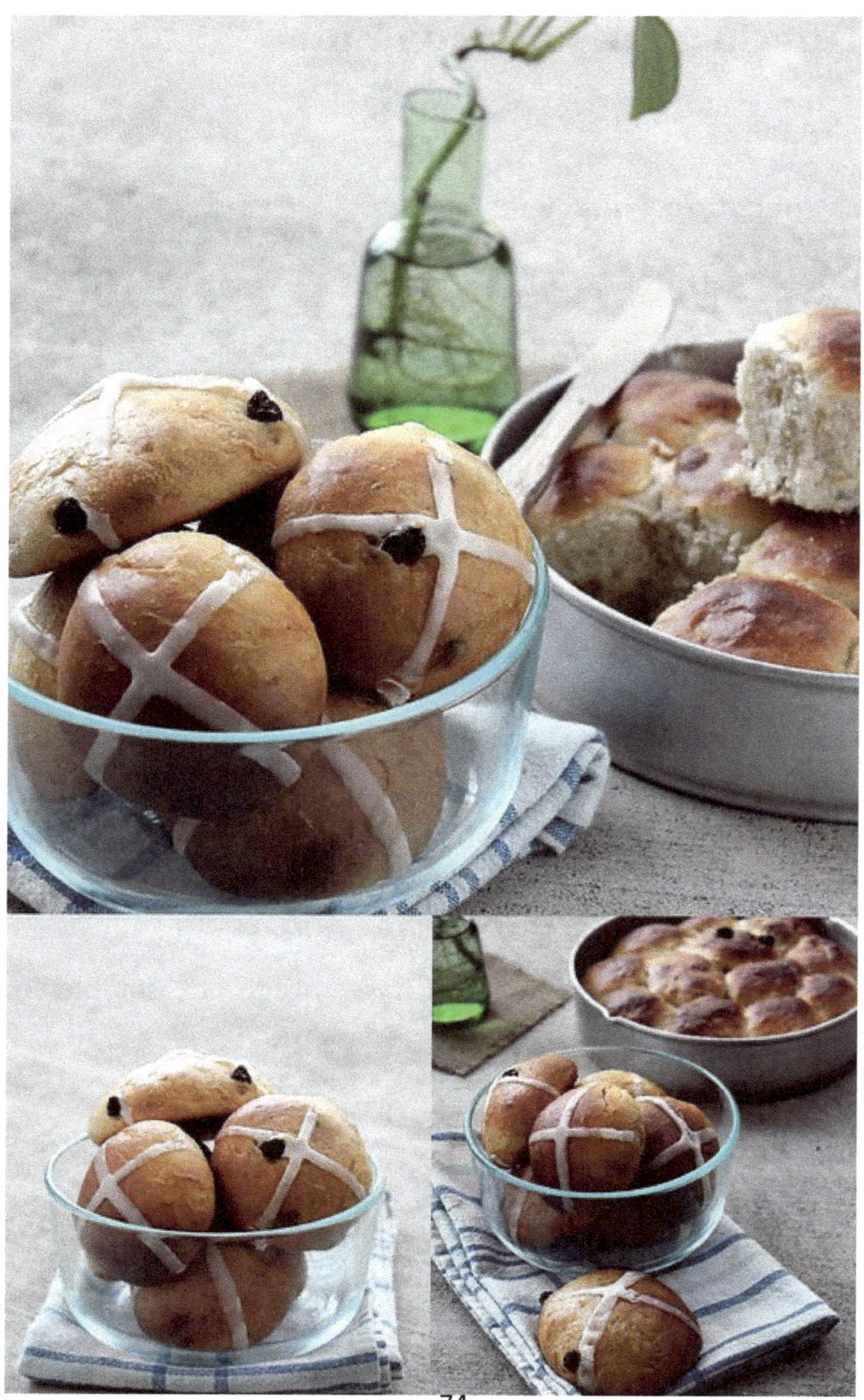

Keto-Friendly Doughnut Recipe

Serves: 4

Cooking Time: 20 minutes

Ingredients:

- ¼ cup coconut milk /62.5ML
- ¼ cup erythritol /32.5G
- ¼ cup flaxseed meal /32.5G
- ¾ cup almond flour /98G
- 1 tablespoon powdered cocoa /15G
- 1 teaspoon vanilla flavor /5ML
- 2 large eggs, beaten
- 3 tablespoons coconut oil /45ML

Instructions:

1) Place all ingredients in the mixing bowl.
2) Mix until well-combined.
3) Scoop the dough into individual doughnut molds.
4) Preheat the air fryer for 5 minutes.
5) Cook for 20 minutes at 350° F or 177°C .
6) Bake in batches if possible.

Nutrition information:

- Calories per serving: 222
- Carbohydrates: 5.1g

- Protein: 3.9g
- Fat: 20.7g

Lava Cake in A Mug

Serves: 4

Cooking Time: 15 minutes

Ingredients:

- ¼ cup coconut oil, melted /62.5ML
- ¼ teaspoon vanilla powder /1.25G
- 1 cup chocolates powder /130G
- 1 tablespoon almond flour /15G
- 2 tablespoons stevia powder /30G
- 3 large eggs, beaten

Instructions:

1) Preheat the air fryer for 5 minutes.
2) Combine all ingredients in a mixing bowl.
3) Grease pan with coconut oil and dust with chocolate powder.
4) Pour the batter in the ramekins and place with the fryer basket.
5) Close and bake at 375° F or 191°C for 15 minutes.

Nutrition information:

- Calories per serving: 251
- Carbohydrates: 14.5g
- Protein: 4.1g

- Fat: 19.6g

Leche Flan Filipino Style

Servings per Recipe: 4

Cooking Time: 30 Minutes

Ingredients:

- 1 cup heavy cream /250ML
- 1 teaspoon vanilla flavor /5ML
- 1/2 (14 ounces) can sweetened condensed milk /420ML
- 1/2 cup milk /125ML
- 2-1/2 eggs
- 1/3 cup white sugar /43G

Instructions:

1) Blend vanilla, eggs, milk, cream, and condensed milk in a blender.
2) Grease baking pan of air fryer with cooking spray. Add sugar and warm for 10 minutes at 370° F or 188°C until melted and caramelized. Lower heat to 300° F or 149°C and continue melting and twirling.
3) Pour milk mixture into caramelized sugar. Cover pan with foil.
4) Cook for 20 minutes at 330° F or 166°C .
5) Allow to cool completely inside a fridge.
6) Place a plate on the pan and invert the pan to easily remove the flan.

7) Serve and enjoy.

Nutrition Information:

- Calories per Serving: 498
- Carbs: 46.8g
- Protein: 10.0g
- Fat: 30.0g

Lusciously Easy Brownies

Servings per Recipe: 8

Cooking Time: 20 minutes

Ingredients:

- 1 egg
- 2 tablespoons and two teaspoons unsweetened cocoa powder /40G
- 1/2 cup white sugar /65G
- 1/2 teaspoon vanilla flavoring /2.5ML
- 1/4 cup butter /32.5G
- 1/4 cup all-purpose flour /32.5G
- 1/8 teaspoon salt /0.625G
- 1/8 teaspoon baking powder /0.625G

- Frosting Ingredients

- 1 tablespoon and 1-1/2 teaspoons butter, softened /22.5G
- 1 tablespoon and 1-1/2 teaspoons unsweetened cocoa powder /22.5G
- 1-1/2 teaspoons honey /7.5ML
- 1/2 teaspoon vanilla flavor /2.5ML
- 1/2 cup confectioners' sugar /65G

Instructions:

1) Grease baking pan of air fryer with cooking spray. Melt ¼ cup butter for 3 minutes. Stir in vanilla, eggs, and sugar. Mix well.
2) Stir in baking powder, salt, flour, and cocoa mix well. Evenly spread.
3) For 20 minutes, cook at 300° F or 149°C .
4) Mix all ingredients in a bowl. Frost brownies while still warm.
5) Serve and enjoy.

Nutrition Information:

- Calories per Serving: 191
- Carbs: 25.7g
- Protein: 1.8g
- Fat: 9.0g

Maple Cinnamon Buns

Serves: 9

Cooking Time: 30 Minutes

Ingredients:

- ¼ cup icing sugar /32.5G
- ½ cup pecan nuts, toasted /65G
- ¾ cup tablespoon unsweetened almond milk /188ML
- 1 ½ cup plain white flour, sifted /195G
- 1 ½ tablespoon active yeast /22.5G
- 1 cup wholegrain flour, sifted /130G
- 1 tablespoon coconut oil, melted /15ML
- 1 tablespoon ground flaxseed /15G
- 2 ripe bananas, sliced
- 2 teaspoons cinnamon powder /10G
- 4 Medjool dates, pitted
- 4 tablespoons maple syrup /60ML

Instructions:

1) Heat ¾ cup almond milk to lukewarm and add the maple syrup and yeast. Allow the yeast to stimulate for 5 to 10 minutes.
2) Mix flaxseed and 3 tablespoons of water to replace eggs. Allow flaxseed to soak for two minutes. Add coconut oil.
3) Pour the flaxseed mixture on the yeast mixture.

4) Mix the 2 kinds of flour and 1 tablespoon cinnamon powder in another bowl. Pour the yeast-flaxseed mixture and combine until dough forms.

5) Knead the dough over a floured flat surface for 10 minutes.

6) Place the kneaded dough in a greased bowl and cover with a kitchen towel. Leave in a dark, warm place for an hour to allow the bread rise.

7) While the dough is rising, mix the pecans, banana slices, and dates. Add 1 tablespoon of cinnamon powder.

8) Preheat the air fryer to 390° F or 199°C .

9) Roll the risen dough on a floured flat surface until it is thin. Spread the pecan mixture on the dough.

10) Roll the dough and cut into nine slices.

11) Place in a dish and cook for 30 minutes.

12) Once cooked, sprinkle with icing sugar.

Nutrition information:

- Calories per serving: 293
- Carbohydrates: 44.9g
- Protein: 5.6g
- Fat:10.1 g

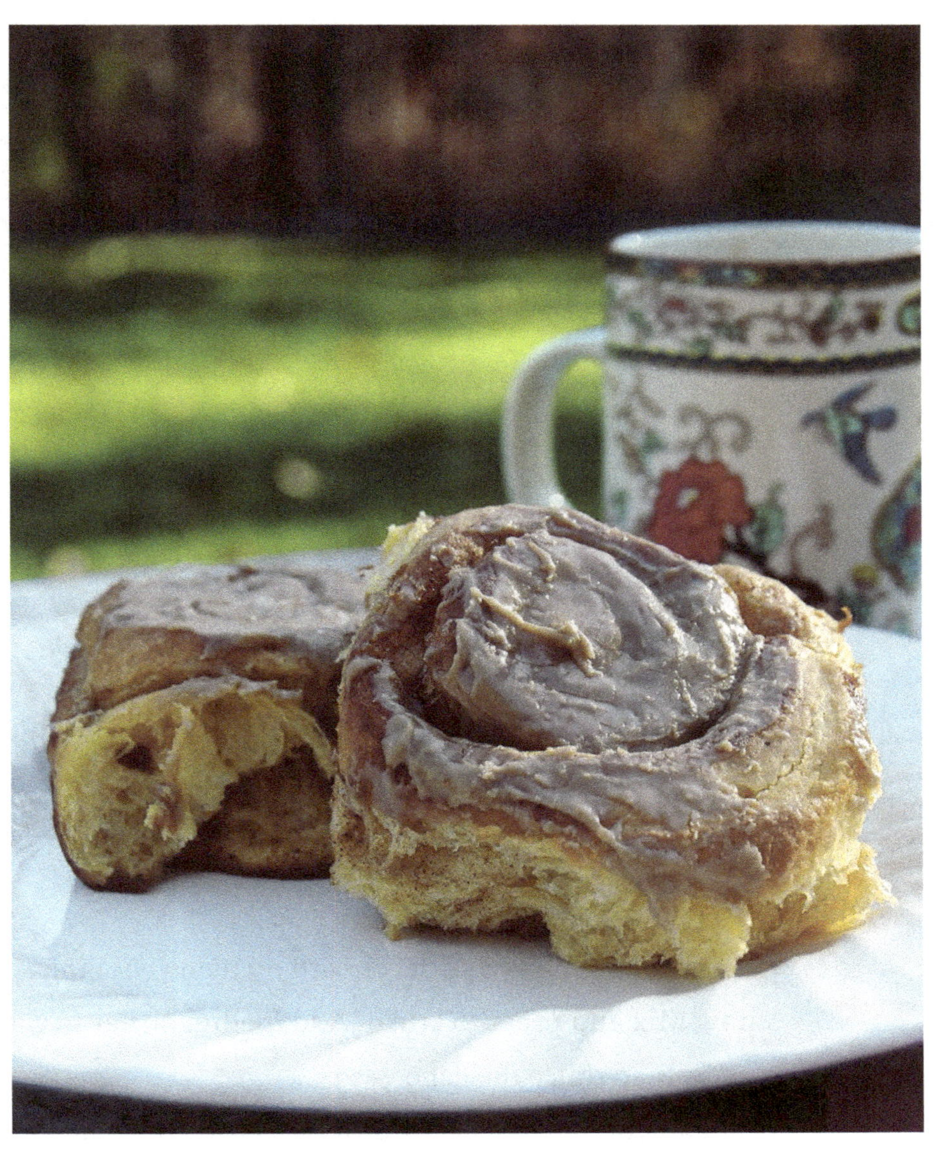

Melts in Your Mouth Caramel Cheesecake

Servings per Recipe: 8

Cooking Time: 40 minutes

Ingredients:

- 1 Can Dulce de Leche
- 1 Tbsp Melted Chocolate /15ML
- 1 Tbsp Vanilla Essence /15ML
- 250 g Caster Sugar
- 4 Large Eggs
- 50 g Melted Butter
- 500 g Soft Cheese
- 6 Digestives, crumbled

Instructions:

1) Grease baking pan of air fryer with oil using cooking spray. Mix and press to crush. Add melted butter to the pan. Spread dulce de leche.
2) Beat soft cheese and sugar until fluffy. Stir in vanilla and egg. Pour mixture over dulce de leche.
3) Cover pan with foil. Cook for 15 minutes at 390° F or 199°C .
4) Reduce to 330° F or 166°C and cook for 10 minutes. Reduce to 300° F or 149°C and cook for 15 minutes.

5) Open the air fryer and allow to cool. After which, place in the refrigerator for 4 hours before slicing.

6) Serve and enjoy.

Nutrition Information:

- Calories per Serving: 463
- Carbs: 44.1g
- Protein: 17.9g
- Fat: 23.8g

Mouth-Watering Strawberry Cobbler

Servings per Recipe: 4

Cooking Time: 25 minutes

Ingredients:

- tablespoon butter, diced /15G
- tablespoon and two teaspoons butter /25G
- 1-1/2 teaspoons cornstarch /7.5G
- 1/2 cup water /125ML
- 1-1/2 cups strawberries, hulled /195G
- 1/2 cup all-purpose flour /65G
- 1-1/2 teaspoons white sugar /7.5G
- 1/4 cup white sugar /32.5G
- 1/4 teaspoon salt /1.25G
- 1/4 cup heavy whipping cream /62.5ML
- 3/4 teaspoon baking powder /3.75G

Instructions:

1) Grease baking pan of air fryer with oil using cooking spray. Add water, cornstarch, and sugar. Cook for 10 minutes at 390° F or 199°C or until hot and thick. Add strawberries and mix well. Dress tops with 1 tbsp butter.

2) Mix salt, baking powder, sugar, and flour. Cut in 1 tbsp and two tsp butter. Mix in cream. Mix in the berries.

3) Cook for 15 minutes at 390° F or 199°C , until tops are
   lightly browned.

4) Serve and enjoy.

Nutrition Information:

- Calories per Serving: 255
- Carbs: 32.0g
- Protein: 2.4g
- Fat: 13.0g

Oriental Coconut Cake

Servings per Recipe: 8

Cooking Time: 40 minutes

Ingredients:

- 1 cup gluten-free flour /130G
- 2 eggs
- 1/2 cup flaked coconut /65G
- 1-1/2 teaspoons baking powder /7.5G
- 1/2 teaspoon baking soda /2.5G
- 1/2 teaspoon xanthan gum /2.5G
- 1/2 teaspoon salt /2.5G
- 1/2 cup coconut milk /125ML
- 1/2 cup vegetable oil /125ML
- 1/2 teaspoon vanilla flavor /2.5ML
- 1/4 cup chopped walnuts /32.5G
- 3/4 cup white sugar /98G

Instructions:

1) Blend all wet ingredients. Add dry ingredients and blend thoroughly.
2) Grease baking pan of air fryer lightly with oil using cooking spray.
3) Pour in batter. Cover pan with foil.
4) Cook for 30 minutes at 330° F or 166°C .

5) Let it rest for 10 Minutes

6) Serve and enjoy.

Nutrition Information:

- Calories per Serving: 359
- Carbs: 35.2g
- Protein: 4.3g
- Fat: 22.3g

Pecan-Cranberry Cake

Servings per Recipe: 6

Cooking Time: 25 minutes

Ingredients:

- 1 1/2 cups Almond Flour /195G
- 1 tsp baking powder /5G
- 1/2 cup fresh cranberries /65G
- 1/2 tsp vanilla extract /2.5ML
- 1/4 cup cashew milk (or use any dairy or non-dairy milk you like) /62.5ML
- 1/4 cup chopped pecans /32.5G
- 1/4 cup Monk fruit (or make use of preferred sweetener) /32.5G
- 1/4 tsp cinnamon /1.25G
- 1/8 tsp salt /0.625G

- 2 large eggs

Instructions:

1) Blend all wet ingredients and mix well. Add all dry ingredients except for cranberries and pecans. Blend well until smooth.
2) Grease baking pan of air fryer with cooking spray. Pour in batter. Sprinkle cranberries and pecans at the top.
3) For twenty minutes, cook on 330° F or 166°C .
4) Allow to sit for 5 minutes.
5) Serve and enjoy

Nutrition Information:

- Calories per Serving: 98
- Carbs: 11.7g
- Protein: 1.7g
- Fat: 4.9g

Poppy Seed Pound Cake

Serves: 8

Cooking Time: 20 Minutes

Ingredients

- ¼ cup erythritol powder /32.5G
- ¼ teaspoon vanilla flavor /1.25ML
- ½ cup coconut milk /125ML
- 1 ½ cups almond flour /195G
- 1 ½ teaspoon baking powder /7.5G
- 1/3 cup butter, unsalted /83G
- 2 large eggs, beaten
- 2 tablespoon psyllium husk powder /30G
- 2 tablespoons poppy seeds /30G

Instructions:

1) Preheat the air fryer for 5 minutes.
2) Combine all ingredients and mix well.
3) Use a hand mixer to mix everything.
4) Pour into a small loaf pan that may easily fit in a mid-air fryer.
5) Bake for 20 minutes at 375° F or 191°C or if a toothpick comes clean after inserted in the middle.

Nutrition information:

- Calories per serving: 145
- Carbohydrates: 3.6
- Protein: 2.1g
- Fat: 13.6g

Pound Cake with Fresh Apples

Servings per Recipe: 6

Cooking Time: 60 minutes

Ingredients

- 1 cup white sugar /250ML
- 1 teaspoon vanilla flavor /5ML
- 1 medium Granny Smith apples - peeled, cored and chopped
- 1-1/2 eggs
- 1-1/2 cups all-purpose flour /195G
- 1/2 teaspoon baking soda /2.5G
- 1/2 teaspoon salt /2.5G
- 1/4 teaspoon ground cinnamon /1.25G
- 2/3 cup and 1 tablespoon chopped walnuts /102G
- 3/4 cup vegetable oil /188ML

Instructions:

1) Blend all ingredients except the apples and walnuts. Blend until smooth. Add apples and walnuts.
2) Lightly grease baking pan of air fryer with cooking spray. Pour batter.
3) Cover pan with foil.
4) Cook for 30 minutes at 330° F or 166°C .

5) Remove foil and cook for another 20 minutes.

6) Let it sit for 10 minutes.

7) Serve and enjoy.

Nutrition Information:

- Calories per Serving: 696
- Carbs: 71.1g
- Protein: 6.5g
- Fat: 42.8g

Quick 'n Easy Pumpkin Pie

Servings per Recipe: 8

Cooking Time: 35 minutes

Ingredients:

- 1 (14 ounces) can sweetened condensed milk /420ML
- 1 (15 ounces) can pumpkin puree /450ML
- 1 9-inch unbaked pie crust
- 1 large egg
- 1 teaspoon ground cinnamon /5G
- 1/2 teaspoon fine salt /2.5G
- 1/2 teaspoon ground ginger / 2.5G
- 1/4 teaspoon freshly grated nutmeg /1.25G
- 1/8 teaspoon Chinese 5-spice powder /0.625G
- 3 egg yolks

Instructions:

1) Lightly grease baking pan of air fryer with oil using cooking spray. Fill the bottom of the pan with pie crust. Puncture with a fork.

2) Blend egg, egg yolks, and pumpkin puree. Add Chinese 5-spice powder, nutmeg, salt, ginger, cinnamon, and condensed milk. Pour on top of pie crust.

3) Cover pan with foil.

4) Cook on preheated 390° F or 199°C air fryer for 15 minutes.

5) Remove foil and continue cooking for 20 minutes at 330° F or 166°C or until the middle is cooked.

6) Allow to cool in the air fryer completely.

7) Serve and enjoy.

Nutrition Information:

- Calories per Serving: 326
- Carbs: 41.9g
- Protein: 7.6g
- Fat: 14.2g

Raspberry-Coco Desert

Serves: 12

Cooking Time: 20 Minutes

Ingredients:

- ¼ cup coconut oil /62.5ML

- 1 cup coconut milk /250ML

- 1 cup raspberries, pulsed /130G

- 1 teaspoon vanilla bean /5G

- 1/3 cup erythritol powder /43G

- 3 cups desiccated coconut /390G

Instructions:

1) Preheat the air fryer for 5 minutes.
2) Combine all ingredients inside a mixing bowl.
3) Pour in a greased baking dish.
4) Bake in the air fryer for 20 minutes at 375° F or 191°C .

Nutrition information:

- Calories per serving: 132

- Carbohydrates: 9.7g

- Protein: 1.5g

- Fat: 9.7g

Raspberry-Coconut Cupcake

Serves: 6

Cooking Time: 30 minutes

Ingredients

- ½ cup butter /65G
- ½ teaspoon salt /2.5G
- ¾ cup erythritol /98G
- 1 cup almond milk, unsweetened /250ML
- 1 cup coconut flour /130G
- 1 tablespoon baking powder /15G
- 3 teaspoons vanilla flavoring /15ML
- 7 large eggs, beaten

Instructions:

1) Preheat air fryer for 5 minutes.
2) Mix all ingredients using a hand mixer.
3) Pour into hard cupcake shapes.
4) Place in the air fryer basket.
5) Bake for 30 minutes at 350° For 177°C or until a toothpick inserted in the middle comes clean.
6) Bake by batches if possible.
7) Allow to chill before serving.

Nutrition information:

- Calories per serving: 235
- Carbohydrates: 7.4g
- Protein: 3.8g
- Fat: 21.1g

Strawberry Pop-Tarts

Servings per Recipe: 6

Cooking Time: 25 minutes

Ingredients:

- 1 oz reduced-fat Philadelphia cream cheese /30G
- 1 tsp cornstarch /5G
- 1 tsp stevia /5G
- 1 tsp sugar sprinkles /5G
- 1/2 cup plain, non-fat vanilla Greek yogurt /125ML
- 1/3 cup low-sugar strawberry preserves /43G
- 2 refrigerated pie crusts
- extra virgin olive oil or coconut oil spray

Instructions:

1) Cut pie crusts into 6 equal rectangles.
2) Mix cornstarch and preserves. Add preserves in the middle of the crust. Fold over crust. Crimp edges with a fork to seal. Repeat the process for the remaining crusts.
3) Lightly grease baking pan of air fryer with cooking spray. Add pop tarts in a single layer. Cook in batches for 8 minutes at 370° F or 188°C .
4) Make frosting by mixing stevia, cream cheese, and yogurt in the bowl. Spread together with a cooked pop tart and add sugar sprinkles.

5) Serve and enjoy.

Nutrition Information:

- Calories per Serving: 317
- Carbs: 34.8g
- Protein: 4.7g
- Fat: 17.6g

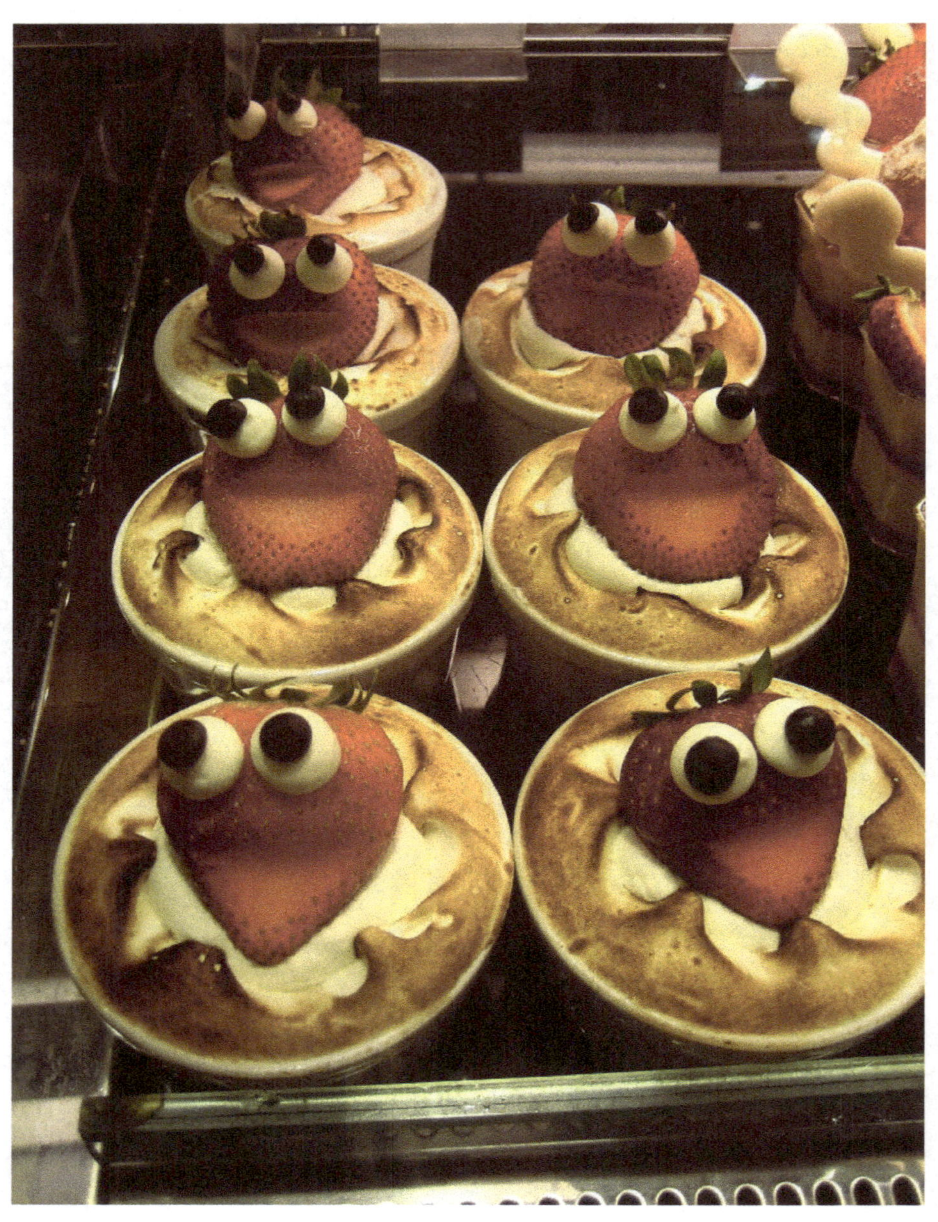

Strawberry Shortcake Quickie

Serves: 4

Cooking Time: 25 minutes

Ingredients:

- ¼ teaspoon liquid stevia /1.25ML
- ¼ teaspoon salt /1.25G
- ½ cup butter /65G
- ½ teaspoon baking powder /2.5G
- 1 cup strawberries, halved /130G
- 1 teaspoon vanilla flavoring /5ML
- 1/3 cup erythritol /43G
- 2/3 cup almond flour /87G
- 3 large eggs, beaten

Instructions:

1) Preheat air fryer for 5 minutes.
2) Combine all ingredients except the strawberries.
3) Use a hand mixer to blend everything.
4) Pour into greased pans
5) Add sliced strawberries to the top
6) Place the pans inside the fryer basket.
7) Bake for 25 minutes at 350° F or 177°C .
8) Place inside the fridge to chill before serving.

Nutrition information:

- Calories per serving: 265
- Carbohydrates: 3.7g
- Protein:2.5 g
- Fat: 26.7g

Vanilla Pound Cake

Serves: 12

Cooking Time: 30 minutes

Ingredients:

- ¼ teaspoon salt /1.25G
- ½ cup erythritol powder /65G
- 1 vanilla bean, scraped
- 1/3 cup water /83ML
- 2/3 cup butter, melted /88ML
- 4 large eggs

Instructions:

1) Preheat air fryer for 5 minutes.
2) Combine all ingredients in the mixing bowl. Mix well.
3) Pour in a greased baking dish.
4) Bake in the air fryer for 30 minutes at 375° F or 191°C.

Nutrition information:

- Calories per serving: 126
- Carbohydrates: 2.3g
- Protein: 1.6g
- Fat: 12.3g

Yummy Banana Cookies

Serves: 6

Cooking Time: 10 minutes

Ingredients:

- 1 cup dates, pitted and chopped /130G
- 1 teaspoon vanilla /5G
- 1/3 cup vegetable oil /83ML
- 2 cups rolled oats /260G
- 3 ripe bananas

Instructions:

1) Preheat the air fryer to 350° F or 177°C .
2) Mash the bananas in a bowl and add the rest of the ingredients.
3) Place in the fridge to marinate for 10 minutes.
4) Drop a teaspoonful on cut parchment paper.
5) Place the cookies on parchment paper inside the air fryer basket. Make sure that the cookies usually do not overlap.
6) Cook for 20 minutes or until the edges are crispy.
7) Serve with almond milk.

Nutrition information:

- Calories per serving: 382

- Carbohydrates: 50.14g
- Protein: 6.54g
- Fat: 17.2g

Zucchini-Choco Bread

Serves: 12

Cooking Time: 20 minutes

Ingredients:

- ¼ teaspoon salt /1.25G
- ½ cup almond milk /125ML
- ½ cup maple syrup /125ML
- ½ cup sunflower oil /125ML
- ½ cup unsweetened powdered cocoa /65G
- 1 cup oat flour /130G
- 1 cup zucchini, shredded and squeezed /250ML
- ·1 tablespoon flax egg (1 tablespoon or 15ML flax meal + 3 tablespoons or 45ML water)
- 1 teaspoon using apple cider vinegar /5ML
- 1 teaspoon baking soda /5G
- 1 teaspoon vanilla extract /5G
- 1/3 cup chocolate chips /43G

Instructions:

1) Preheat the air fryer to 350° F or 177°C .
2) Line a baking dish with wax paper.
3) In a bowl, combine the flax meal, zucchini, sunflower oil, maple, vanilla, apple cider vinegar and milk. Mix well.

4) Add oat flour, baking soda, hot chocolate mix, and salt.
   Mix until well combined.
5) Add the chocolate chips.
6) Pour the mixture inside a baking dish and cook for 15
   minutes or until a toothpick inserted in the middle comes
   out clean.

Nutrition information:

- Calories per serving: 213
- Carbohydrates:24.2 g
- Protein: 4.6g
- Fat: 10.9g